Easy Keto Air Fryer Diet Cookbook

Quick and Easy Seafood Recipes to Boost your Health

Olivia Read

Introduction

What's the difference between an air fryer and deep fryer? Air fryers bake food a high temperature with a high-powered fan, while deep fryers cook food in a vat of oil that has been heated up to a specific temperature. Both cook food quickly, but an air fryer requires practically zero preheat time while a deep fryer can take upwards of 10 minutes. Air fryers also require little to no oil and deep fryers require a lot that absorb into the food. Food comes out crispy and juicy in both appliances, but don't taste the same, usually because deep fried foods are coated in batter that cook differently in an air fryer vs a deep fryer. Battered foods needs to be sprayed with oil before cooking in an air fryer to help them color and get crispy, while the hot oil soaks into the batter in a deep fryer. Flour-based batters and wet batters don't cook well in an air fryer, but they come out very well in a deep fryer.

The ketogenic diet is one such example. The diet calls for a very small number of carbs to be eaten. This means food such as rice, pasta, and other starchy vegetables like potatoes are off the menu. Even relaxed versions of the keto diet minimize carbs to a large extent and this compromises the goals of many dieters. They end up having to exert large amounts of willpower to follow the diet. This doesn't do them any favors since willpower is like a muscle. At some point, it tires and this is when the dieter goes right back to their old pattern of eating. I have personal experience with this. In terms of health benefits, the keto diet offers the most. The reduction of carbs

4

forces your body to mobilize fat and this results in automatic fat loss and better health.

Feel free to mix and match the recipes you see in here and play around with them. Eating is supposed to be fun! Unfortunately, we've associated fun eating with unhealthy food. This doesn't have to be the case. The air fryer, combined with the Mediterranean diet, will make your mealtimes fun-filled again and full of taste. There's no grease and messy cleanups to deal with anymore. Are you excited yet?

You should be! You're about to embark on a journey full of air fried goodness!

Table of Contents

Quick-Fix Seafood Breakfast

Cook Time:

30 minutes

Servings:2

Ingredients

1 tablespoon olive oil
2 garlic cloves, minced
1 small yellow onion, chopped
1/4 pound tilapia pieces
1/4 pound rockfish pieces
1/2 teaspoon dried basil
Salt and white pepper, to taste
4 eggs, lightly beaten
1 tablespoon dry sherry
4 tablespoons cheese, shredded

Directions:

1.Start by preheating your Air Fryer to 350 degrees F; add the olive oil to a baking pan.

2.Once hot, cook the garlic and onion for 2 minutes or until fragrant.

3.Add the fish, basil, salt, and pepper. In a mixing dish, thoroughly combine the eggs with sherry and cheese. Pour the mixture into the baking pan.

4.Cook at 360 degrees F approximately 20 minutes. Serve and enjoy!

8

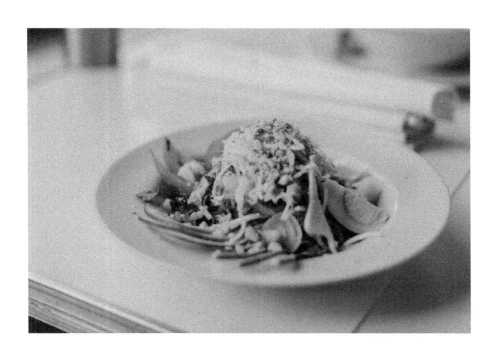

Grilled Hake with Garlic Sauce

Cooking Time:

30 minutes

Servings:3

Ingredients:

3hake fillets
6tablespoons mayonnaise
1 teaspoon Dijon mustard
1 tablespoon fresh lime juice
1 cup panko crumbs
Salt, to taste
1/4 teaspoon ground black pepper, or more to taste

Garlic Sauce:

1/4 cup Greek-style yogurt

2 tablespoons olive oil

2 cloves garlic, minced

1/2 teaspoon tarragon leaves, minced

Directions:

1.Pat dry the hake fillets with a kitchen towel. In a shallow bowl, whisk together the mayo, mustard, and lime juice.

2.In another shallow bowl, thoroughly combine the panko crumbs with salt, and black pepper. Spritz the Air Fryer grill pan with non-stick cooking spray.

3.Grill in the preheated Air Fry at 395 degrees F for 10 minutes, flipping halfway through the cooking time. Serve immediately.

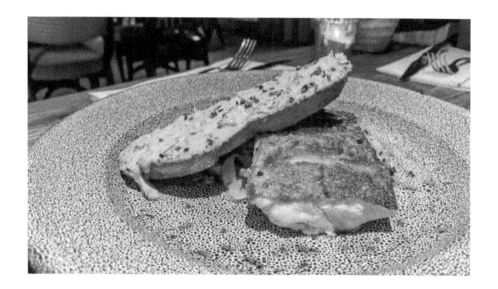

Buttermilk Tuna fillets

Cooking Time:

35 minutes

Servings:3

Ingredients:

1pound tuna fillets

1/2 cup buttermilk

1/2 cup tortilla chips, crushed

1/4 cup parmesan cheese, grated

1/4 cup cassava flour

Salt and ground black pepper, to taste

1 teaspoon mustard seeds

1 teaspoon paprika

1 teaspoon garlic powder

1/2 teaspoon onion powder

Directions:

1.Place the tuna fillets and buttermilk in a bowl; cover and let it sit for 30 minutes.

2.In a shallow bowl, thoroughly combine the remaining ingredients; mix until well combined.

3.Dip the tuna fillets in the parmesan mixture until they are covered on all sides. Cook in the preheated Air Fryer at 380 degrees F for 12 minutes, turning halfway through the cooking time. Serve and enjoy!

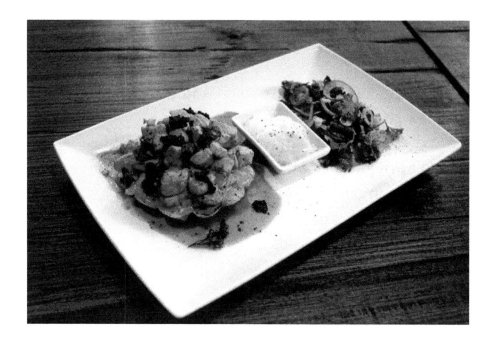

King Prawns with Lemon Butter Sauce

Cooking Time:

15 minutes

Servings:4

Ingredients:

King Prawns:

1 ½ pounds king prawns, peeled and deveined

2 cloves garlic, minced

1/2 cup Pecorino Romano cheese, grated

Sea salt and ground white pepper, to your liking

1/2 teaspoon onion powder

1teaspoon garlic powder

1teaspoon mustard seeds

1tablespoons olive oil

Sauce:

2 tablespoons butter

2 tablespoons fresh lemon juice

1/2 teaspoon Worcestershire sauce

1/4 teaspoon ground black pepper

Directions:

1.In a plastic closeable bag, thoroughly combine all ingredients for the king prawns; shake to combine well.

2.Transfer the coated king prawns to the lightly greased Air Fryer basket.

3.Cook in the preheated Air Fryer at 390 degrees for 6 minutes, shaking the basket halfway through. Work in batches.

4.In the meantime, heat a small saucepan over a moderate flame; melt the butter and add the remaining ingredients.

5.Turn the temperature to low and whisk for 2 to 3 minutes until thoroughly heated. Spoon the sauce onto the warm king prawns. Serve and enjoy!

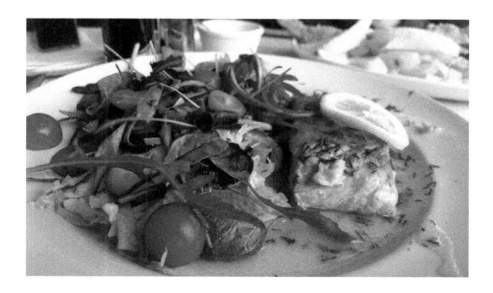

Sea Bass with French Sauce Tartare

Cooking Time:

15 minutes

Servings:2

Ingredients:

1tablespoon olive oil

2 sea bass fillets

Sauce:

1/2 cup mayonnaise

1 tablespoon capers, drained and chopped

1 tablespoon gherkins, drained and chopped

2 tablespoons scallions, finely chopped

2 tablespoons lemon juice

Directions:

1.Start by preheating your Air Fryer to 395 degrees F. Drizzle olive oil all over the fish fillets.

2.Cook the sea bass in the preheated Air Fryer for 10 minutes, flipping them halfway through the cooking time.

3.Meanwhile, make the sauce by whisking the remaining ingredients until everything is well incorporated. Place in the refrigerator until ready to serve. Enjoy!

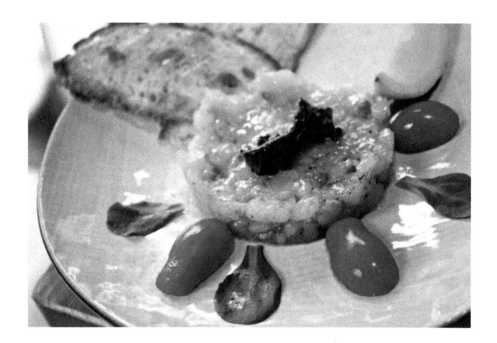

Rosemary-Infused Butter Scallops

Cook Time:

1 hour 10

minutes

Servings:4

Ingredients:

1pounds sea scallops

1/2 cup beer

4 tablespoons butter

2 sprigs rosemary, only leaves

Sea salt and freshly cracked black pepper, to taste

Directions:

1.In a ceramic dish, mix the sea scallops with beer; let it marinate for 1 hour. Meanwhile, preheat your Air Fryer to 400 degrees F.

2.Melt the butter and add the rosemary leaves. Stir for a few minutes. Discard the marinade and transfer the sea scallops to the Air Fryer basket.

3.Season with salt and black pepper. Cook the scallops in the preheated Air Fryer for 7 minutes, shaking the basket halfway through the cooking time. Work in batches.

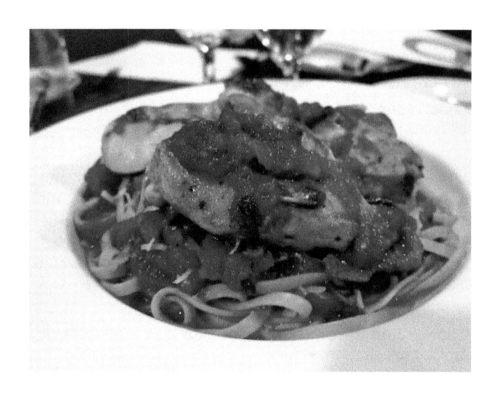

Greek Sardeles Psites

Cooking Time:

40 minutes

Servings:2

Ingredients:

1/4 teaspoon chili paper flakes

Directions:

1.Coat your sardines with all-purpose flour until well coated on all sides.

2.Season your sardines with salt and black pepper and arrange them in the cooking basket. Cook in your Air Fryer at 325 degrees F for 35 to 40 minutes until the skin is crispy.

3.Meanwhile, heat olive oil in a frying pan over a moderate flame.

4.Now, sauté the onion and garlic for 4 to 5 minutes or until tender and aromatic.

5.Stir in the remaining ingredients, cover and let it simmer, for about 15 minutes or until the sauce has thickened and reduced.

6.Spoon the sauce over the warm sardines and serve immediately. Enjoy!

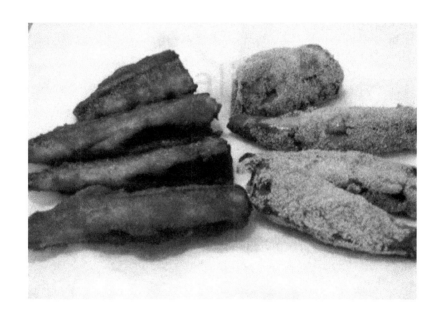

Halibut Steak with Cremini Mushrooms

Cooking Time:

15 minutes

Servings:4

Ingredients:

pound halibut steak

1 teaspoon olive oil

Sea salt and ground black pepper, to taste

6ounces Cremini mushrooms

1 teaspoon butter, melted

1/4 teaspoon onion powder

1/4 teaspoon garlic powder

1/2 teaspoon rosemary

1/2 teaspoon basil

1/2 teaspoon oregano

Directions:

1.Toss the halibut steak with olive oil, salt and black pepper and transfer to the Air Fryer cooking basket.

3.Toss the Cremini mushrooms with the other ingredients until well coated on all sides. Cook the halibut steak at 400 degrees F for 5 minutes.

4.Turn the halibut steak over and top with mushrooms. Continue to cook an additional 5 minutes or until the mushrooms are fragrant. Serve warm and enjoy!

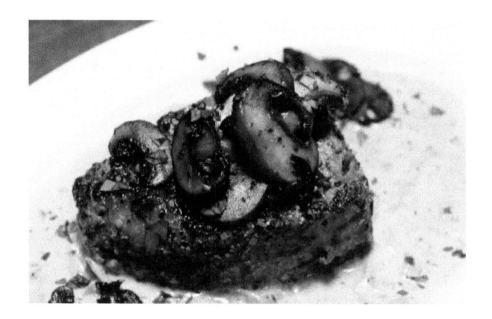

Haddock Steaks with Decadent Mango Salsa

Cooking Time:

15 minutes

Servings:2

Ingredients:

1haddock steaks

1 teaspoon butter, melted

1 tablespoon white wine

Sea salt and ground black pepper, to taste

Mango salsa:

1/2 mango, diced

1/4 cup red onion, chopped

1 chili pepper, deveined and minced

1 teaspoon cilantro, chopped

2 tablespoons fresh lemon juice

Directions:

1.Toss the haddock with butter, wine, salt and black pepper.

2.Cook the haddock in your Air Fryer at 400 degrees F for 5 minutes. Flip the haddock and cook on the other side for 5 minutes more.

3.Meanwhile, make the mango salsa by mixing all ingredients. Serve the warm haddock with the chilled mango salsa and enjoy!

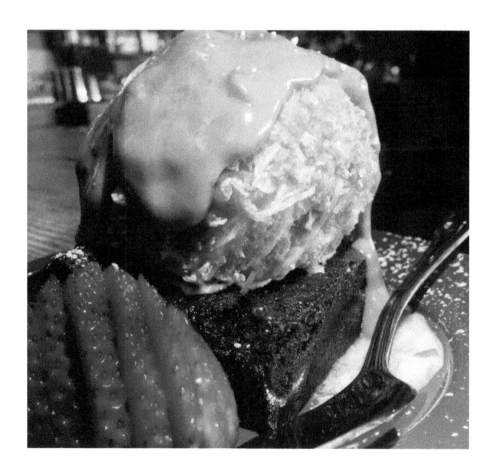

Halibut Steak with Zoodles and Lemon

Cooking Time:

15 minutes

Servings:3

Ingredients:

1pound halibut steak, cut into

3 pieces

1 garlic clove, halved

1 teaspoon avocado oil

Sea salt and black pepper, to taste

1 pound zucchini, julienned

1/2 teaspoon onion powder

1/2 teaspoon granulated garlic

1 tablespoon fresh parsley, minced

1 teaspoon sage, minced

1 lemon, sliced

Directions:

1.Rub the halibut steaks with garlic and toss with avocado oil, salt and black pepper; then, transfer the halibut steaks to the Air Fryer cooking basket.

2.Cook the halibut steak at 400 degrees F for 5 minutes.

3.Turn the halibut steak over and continue to cook an additional 5 minutes or until it flakes easily when tested with a fork.

4.Meanwhile, spritz a wok with a nonstick spray; heat the wok over medium-high heat. Once hot, stir fry the zucchini noodles

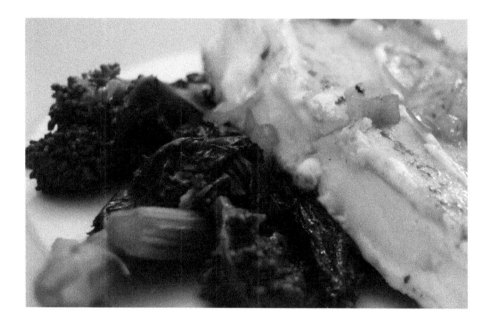

Saucy Garam Masala Fish

Cook Time:

25 minutes

Servings:2

Ingredients:

1teaspoons olive oil

1/4 cup coconut milk

1/2 teaspoon cayenne pepper

1 teaspoon Garam masala

1/4 teaspoon Kala namak Indian black salt

1/2 teaspoon fresh ginger, grated

1 garlic clove, minced

2 catfish fillets

1/4 cup coriander, roughly chopped

Directions:

1.Preheat your Air Fryer to 390 degrees F. Then, spritz the baking dish with a nonstick cooking spray.

2.In a mixing bowl, whisk the olive oil, milk, cayenne pepper, Garam masala, Kala namak, ginger, and garlic.

3.Coat the catfish fillets with the Garam masala mixture. Cook the catfish fillets in the preheated Air Fryer approximately 18 minutes, turning over halfway through the cooking time.

4.Garnish with fresh coriander and serve over hot noodles if desired. Enjoy!

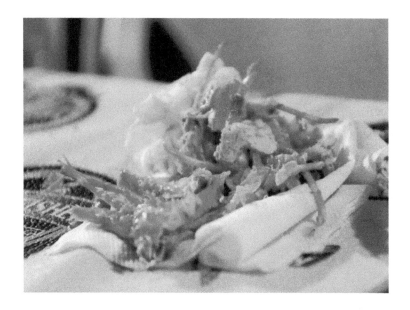

Old Bay Shrimp

Preparation Time:

10 minutes

Cooking Time:

10 minutes

Serve: 4

Ingredients:

12 oz shrimp, peeled
3/25 oz pork rind, crushed
1 1/2 tsp old bay seasoning
1/4 cup mayonnaise

Directions:

1.In a shallow bowl, mix together crushed pork rind and old bay seasoning.

2.Add shrimp and mayonnaise into the mixing bowl and toss well. Place the cooking tray in the air fryer basket. Select Air Fry mode.

3.Set time to 10 minutes and temperature 380 F then press START. The air fryer display will prompt you to ADD FOOD once the temperature is reached then coat shrimp with crushed pork rind and place in the air fryer basket. Serve and enjoy.

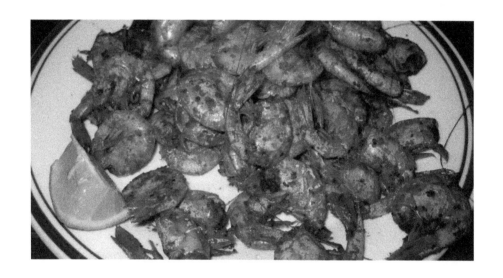

Garlic Butter Fish Fillets

Preparation Time:

10 minutes

Cooking Time:

10 minutes

Serve: 2

Ingredients:

2 salmon fillets
1/4 tsp dried parsley
1 tsp garlic, minced
2 tbsp butter, melted
Pepper Salt

Directions:

1.In a small bowl, mix together melted butter, garlic, and parsley.

2.Season fish fillets with pepper and salt and brush with melted butter mixture.

3.Place the cooking tray in the air fryer basket. Select Air Fry mode. Set time to 10 minutes and temperature 360 F then press START.

4.The air fryer display will prompt you to ADD FOOD once the temperature is reached then place fish fillets skin side down in the air fryer basket. Serve and enjoy.

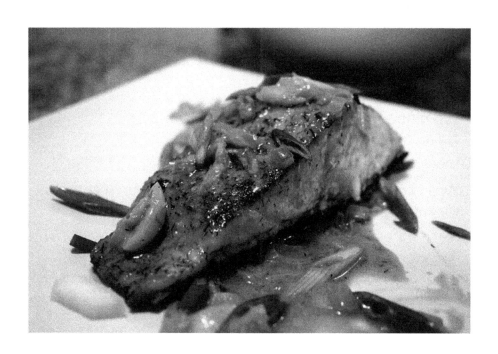

Flavorful Tuna Steaks

Preparation Time:

10 minutes

Cooking Time:

4 minutes

Serve: 2

Ingredients:

12 tuna steaks, skinless and boneless
1/2 tsp rice vinegar
1 tsp sesame oil
1 tsp ginger, grated
4 tbsp soy sauce

Directions:

1.Add tuna steaks and remaining ingredients in the zip-lock bag.

2.Seal bag and place in the refrigerator for 30 minutes. Select Air Fry mode. Set time to 4 minutes and temperature 380 F then press START.

3.The air fryer display will prompt you to ADD FOOD once the temperature is reached then place marinated tuna steaks in the air fryer basket. Serve and enjoy.

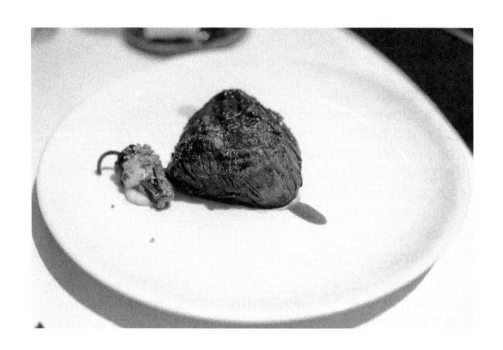

Baked Parmesan Tilapia

Preparation Time:

10 minutes

Cooking Time:

10 minutes

Serve: 4

Ingredients:

2 lbs tilapia
1/4 tsp paprika
1/4 tsp dried basil
2 garlic cloves, minced
1 tsp dried parsley
1 tbsp butter, softened
2tbsp fresh lemon juice
1/4 cup mayonnaise
1/2 cup parmesan cheese, grated
1/2 tsp salt

Directions:

1.In a small bowl, mix together parmesan cheese, mayonnaise, lemon juice, butter, parsley, garlic, basil, paprika, and salt.

2.Place the cooking tray in the air fryer basket. Line air fryer basket with parchment paper. Select Bake mode. Set time to 10 minutes and temperature 400 F then press START.

3.The air fryer display will prompt you to ADD FOOD once the temperature is reached then place fish fillets in the air fryer basket and spread the parmesan mixture on top of each fish fillet. Serve and enjoy.

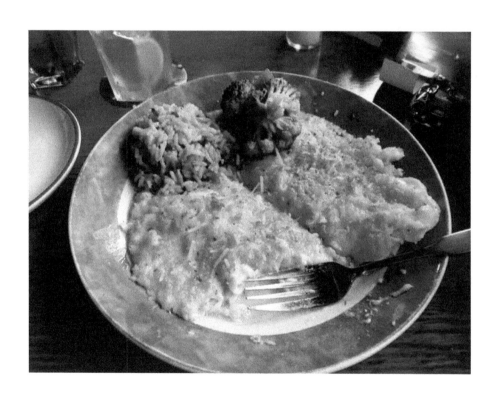

Bagel Crust Fish Fillets

Preparation Time:

10 minutes

Cooking Time:

10 minutes

Serve: 4

Ingredients:

4 white fish fillets
1 tbsp mayonnaise
1 tsp lemon pepper seasoning
2 tbsp almond flour
1/4 cup bagel seasoning

Directions:

1.In a small bowl, mix together bagel seasoning, almond flour, and lemon pepper seasoning. Brush mayonnaise over fish fillets.

2.Sprinkle seasoning mixture over fish fillets. Place the cooking tray in the air fryer basket. Line air fryer basket with parchment paper.

3.Select Bake mode. Set time to 10 minutes and temperature 400 F then press START.

4.The air fryer display will prompt you to ADD FOOD once the temperature is reached then place fish fillets in the air fryer basket. Serve and enjoy.

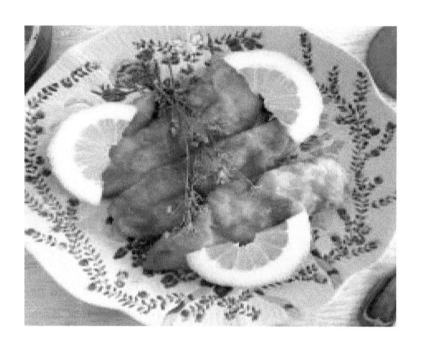

Baked Salmon Patties

Preparation Time:

10 minutes

Cooking Time:

20 minutes

Serve: 4

Ingredients:

2 eggs, lightly beaten
12 oz can salmon, skinless, boneless, and drained
1/2 cup almond flour
1/2 tsp pepper
1tbsp Dijon mustard
1 tsp garlic powder
2 tbsp fresh parsley, chopped
1/2 cup celery, diced
1/2 cup bell pepper, diced
1/2 cup onion, diced

Directions:

1.Add salmon and remaining ingredients into the mixing bowl and mix until well combined.

2.Make 8 equal shapes of patties from the mixture. Place the cooking tray in the air fryer basket. Line air fryer basket with parchment paper.

3.Select Bake mode. Set time to 20 minutes and temperature 400 F then press START.

4.The air fryer display will prompt you to ADD FOOD once the temperature is reached then place patties in the air fryer basket. Turn patties halfway through. Serve and enjoy.

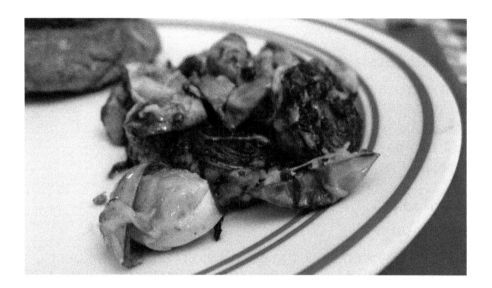

Pesto Scallops

Preparation Time:

10 minutes

Cooking Time:

10minutes

Serve: 4

Ingredients:

1 lb sea scallops
2 tsp garlic, minced
3 tbsp heavy cream
1/4 cup basil pesto
1 tbsp olive oil
1/2 tsp pepper
1 tsp salt

Directions:

1.In a small pan, mix together oil, cream, garlic, pesto, pepper, and salt, and simmer for 2-3 minutes. Select Air Fry mode.

2.Set time to 5 minutes and temperature 320 F then press START.

3.The air fryer display will prompt you to ADD FOOD once the temperature is reached then add scallops in the air fryer basket.

4.Turn scallops and after 3 minutes. Transfer scallops into the mixing bowl. Pour pesto sauce over scallops and serve.

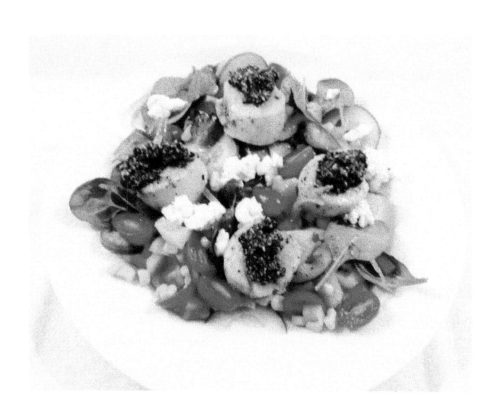

Juicy Baked Halibut

Preparation Time:

10 minutes

Cooking Time:

12 minutes

Serve: 4

Ingredients:

1lb halibut fillets

1/4 tsp garlic powder

1/4 tsp paprika

1/4 tsp pepper

1/4 cup olive oil

1 lemon juice

1/2 tsp salt

Directions:
1.In a small bowl, mix together olive oil, lemon juice, pepper, paprika, garlic powder, and salt.

2.Brush olive oil mixture over fish fillets. Place the cooking tray in the air fryer basket. Line air fryer basket with parchment paper.

3.Select Bake mode. Set time to 12 minutes and temperature 400 F then press START.

4.The air fryer display will prompt you to ADD FOOD once the temperature is reached then place fish fillets in the air fryer basket. Serve and enjoy

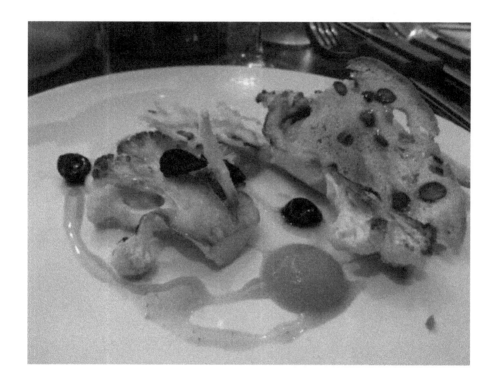

Simple Salmon Patties

Preparation Time:

10 minutes

Cooking Time:

14 minutes

Serve: 4

Ingredients:

1eggs, lightly beaten

2 oz salmon, cooked and flaked

1/4 tsp paprika

1/8 tsp pepper

1/3 cup parsley, chopped

2 garlic cloves, minced

1/4 cup onion, diced

2/3 cup almond flour

Pinch of salt

Directions:

1.Add all ingredients into the mixing bowl and mix until well combined. Make the equal shape of patties from the mixture.

2.Place the cooking tray in the air fryer basket. Line air fryer basket with parchment paper. Select Air Fry mode.

3.Set time to 14 minutes and temperature 380 F then press START.

4.The air fryer display will prompt you to ADD FOOD once the temperature is reached then place patties in the air fryer basket.

5.Turn patties halfway through. Serve and enjoy.

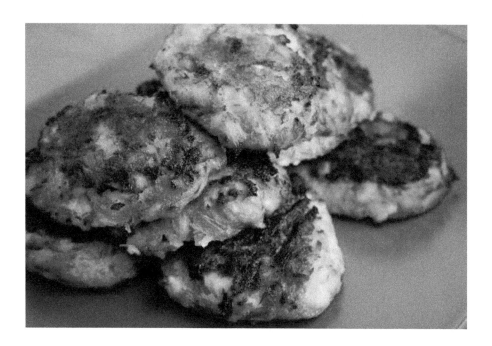

Baked Mahi Mahi

Preparation Time:

10 minutes

Cooking Time:

30 minutes

Serve: 4

Ingredients:

4 Mahi Mahi fillets
1 tsp onion powder
1 tsp garlic powder
1 tsp turmeric
1 tbsp dried basil
1 tsp pepper
1 tsp salt

Directions:

1.In a small bowl, mix together onion powder, garlic powder, turmeric, basil, pepper, and salt. Season fish fillets with spice mixture.

2.Place the cooking tray in the air fryer basket. Line air fryer basket with parchment paper.

3.Select Bake mode. Set time to 30 minutes and temperature 350 F then press START.

4.The air fryer display will prompt you to ADD FOOD once the temperature is reached then place the fish fillet in the air fryer basket. Serve and enjoy.

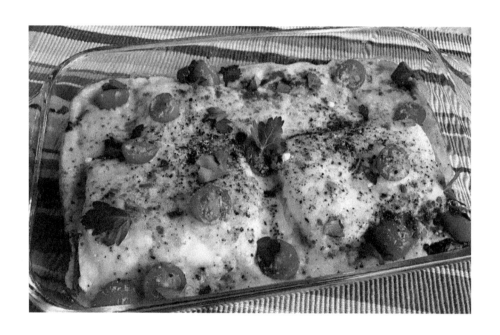

Parmesan Cod

Preparation Time:

10 minutes

Cooking Time:

15 minutes

Serve: 4

Ingredients:

4 cod fillets
1 tbsp olive oil
1 tbsp parsley, chopped
2 tsp paprika
3/4 cup parmesan cheese, grated
1/4 tsp sea salt

Directions:

1.In a shallow dish, mix together parmesan cheese, paprika, parsley, and salt.

2.Brush fish fillets with oil and coat with cheese mixture. Place the cooking tray in the air fryer basket. Line air fryer basket with parchment paper.

3.Select Bake mode. Set time to 15 minutes and temperature 400 F then press START.

4.The air fryer display will prompt you to ADD FOOD once the temperature is reached then place the fish fillet in the air fryer basket. Serve and enjoy.

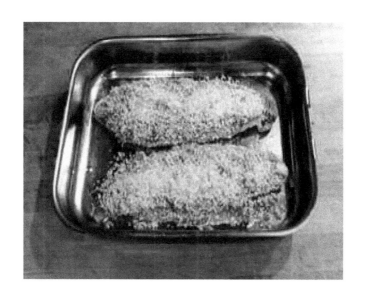

Baked Mayo Cod

Preparation Time:

10 minutes

Cooking Time:

10 minutes

Serve: 4

Ingredients:

4 cod fillets
1/2 cup almond flour
1 tbsp parsley, chopped
1/2 tsp old bay seasoning
1/2 tsp lemon zest
1 tbsp lemon juice
1/4 cup parmesan cheese, grated
1/4 cup onion, minced
2 tbsp butter, melted
1/3 cup mayonnaise

Directions:

1.In a bowl, mix together mayonnaise, butter, onion, cheese, lemon juice, lemon zest, old bay seasoning, and parsley.

2.Spread mayonnaise mixture on top of fish fillets. Sprinkle with almond flour. Place the cooking tray in the air fryer basket.

3.Line air fryer basket with parchment paper. Select Bake mode. Set time to 10 minutes and temperature 400 F then press START.

4.The air fryer display will prompt you to ADD FOOD once the temperature is reached then place the fish fillet in the air fryer basket. Serve and enjoy.

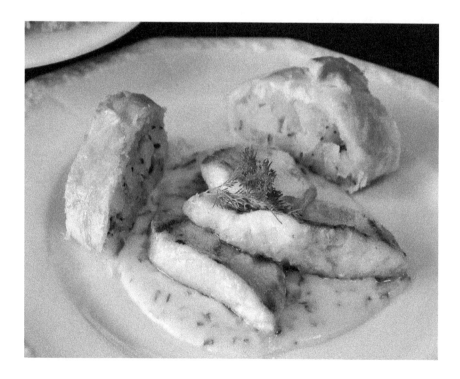

Lemon Pepper Tilapia

Preparation Time:

10 minutes

Cooking Time:

15 minutes

Serve: 4

Ingredients:

4 tilapia fillets, thawed
4 tbsp lemon pepper seasoning

Directions:

1.Spray fish fillets with cooking spray. Sprinkle lemon pepper seasoning over fish fillets. Place the cooking tray in the air fryer basket.

2.Line air fryer basket with parchment paper. Select Bake mode. Set time to 15 minutes and temperature 350 F then press START.

3.The air fryer display will prompt you to ADD FOOD once the temperature is reached then place the fish fillet in the air fryer basket. Serve and enjoy.

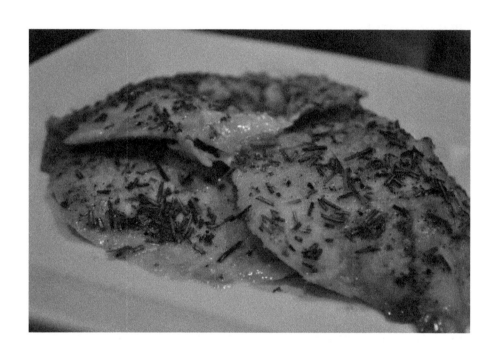

Cajun Salmon Cakes

Preparation Time:

10 minutes

Cooking Time:

15 minutes

Serve: 4

Ingredients:

2 eggs, lightly beaten
12 oz can salmon, boneless & skinless
3/4 cup almond flour
2 1/2 tsp Cajun seasoning
1/2 onion, chopped
1/2 bell pepper, chopped
2 tbsp mayonnaise
Pepper Salt

Directions:

1.Add all ingredients into the mixing bowl and mix until well combined.

2.Make 8 equal shapes of patties from the mixture. Place the cooking tray in the air fryer basket. Line air fryer basket with parchment paper.

3.Select Bake mode. Set time to 10 minutes and temperature 375 F then press START.

4.The air fryer display will prompt you to ADD FOOD once the temperature is reached then add patties in the air fryer basket. Broil patties for 5 minutes.

5.Serve and enjoy.

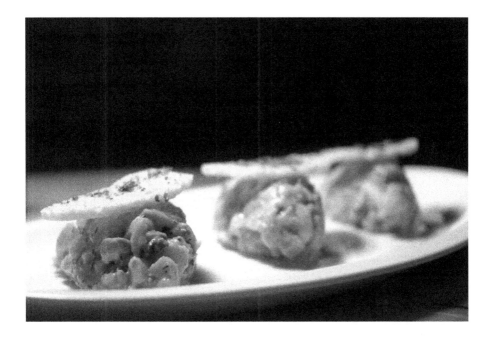

Creamy Spinach

Preparation Time:

10 minutes

Cooking Time:

20 minutes

Serve: 6

Ingredients:

1lb fresh spinach

1 tbsp onion, minced

8 oz cream cheese

6 oz gouda cheese, shredded

1 tsp garlic powder

Pepper Salt

Directions:

1.Spray a large pan with cooking spray and heat over medium heat. Add spinach to the pan and cook until wilted.

2.Add cream cheese, garlic powder, and onion and stir until cheese is melted. Remove pan from heat and add Gouda cheese and season with pepper and salt.

3.Transfer spinach mixture into the greased baking dish. Select Bake mode. Set time to 20 minutes and temperature 400 F then press START.

4.The air fryer display will prompt you to ADD FOOD once the temperature is reached then place the baking dish in the air fryer basket. Serve and enjoy.

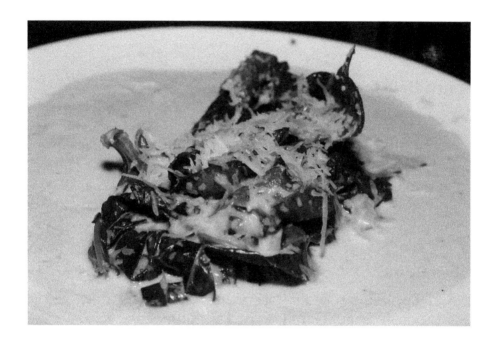

Broccoli Nuggets

Preparation Time:

10 minutes

Cooking Time:

20 minutes

Serve: 4

Ingredients:

1cups broccoli florets, cooked until soften

1/4 cup almond flour

2 egg whites

1 cup cheddar cheese, shredded

1/8 tsp salt

Directions:

1.Add cooked broccoli florets into the large bowl and using potato masher mash into small pieces.

2.Add remaining ingredients into the bowl and mix until well combined. Make small nuggets from the broccoli mixture. Select Bake mode.

3.Set time to 20 minutes and temperature 350 F then press START. The air fryer display will prompt you to ADD FOOD once the temperature is reached then place broccoli nuggets in the air fryer basket.

4.Serve and enjoy.

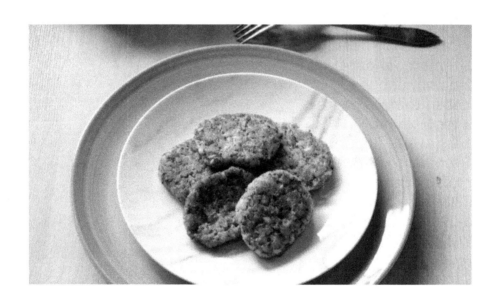

Cauliflower Tomato Rice

Preparation Time:

10 minutes

Cooking Time:

15 minutes

Serve: 3

Ingredients:

1 cauliflower head, cut into florets
1 tomato, chopped
1 onion, chopped
2 tbsp tomato paste
2 tbsp olive oil
1 tsp white pepper
1 tsp black pepper
1 tbsp dried thyme
2 chilies, chopped
2 garlic cloves, chopped
1/2 tsp salt

Directions:

1.Add cauliflower florets into the food processor and process until it looks like rice. Stir in tomato paste, tomatoes, and spices and mix well.

2.Spread cauliflower mixture into the baking dish and drizzle with olive oil.

3Select Bake mode. Set time to 15 minutes and temperature 400 F then press START.

4.The air fryer display will prompt you to ADD FOOD once the temperature is reached then place the baking dish in the air fryer basket. Serve and enjoy.

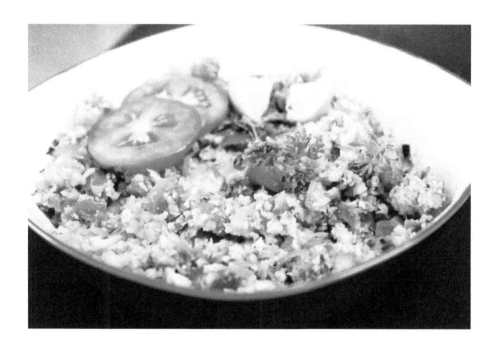

Cheesy Zucchini Noodles

Preparation Time:

10 minutes

Cooking Time:

45 minutes

Serve: 3

Ingredients:

1 egg
2 medium zucchini, trimmed and spiralized
1/2 cup parmesan cheese, grated
1/2 cup feta cheese, crumbled
2 tbsp olive oil
1 cup mozzarella cheese, grated
1 tbsp thyme
1 garlic clove, chopped
1 onion, chopped
1/2 tsp pepper
1/2 tsp salt

Directions:

1.Add spiralized zucchini and salt in a colander and set aside for 10 minutes.

2.Gently wash zucchini noodles and pat dry with a paper towel.

3.Heat oil in a pan over medium heat. Add garlic and onion and sauté for 3-4 minutes. Add zucchini noodles and cook for 4 minutes or until softened.

4.Add zucchini mixture into a baking dish add the eggs, thyme, cheeses. Mix well and season with pepper and salt.

5.Select Bake mode. Set time to 45 minutes and temperature 375 F then press START.

6.The air fryer display will prompt you to ADD FOOD once the temperature is reached then place the baking dish in the air fryer basket. Serve and enjoy.

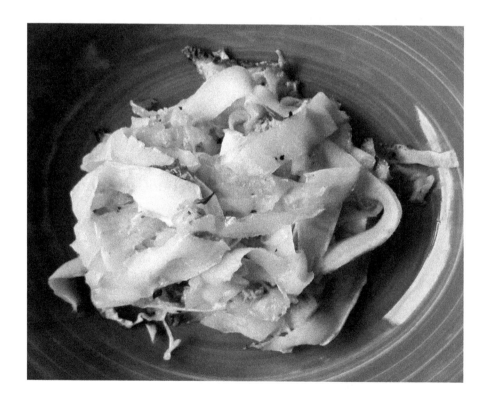

Cheese Baked Broccoli

Preparation Time:

10 minutes

Cooking Time:

10 minutes

Serve: 4

Ingredients:

1 lb broccoli, cut into florets
1/2 cup mozzarella cheese, shredded
1/2 cup heavy cream
2 garlic cloves, minced
1/4 cup parmesan cheese, grated
1/2 cup gruyere cheese, shredded
1 tbsp butter

Directions:

1.Melt butter in a pan over medium heat. Add broccoli and season with pepper and salt.

2.Cook broccoli over medium heat for 5 minutes or until tender.

3.Add garlic and stir for a minute. Transfer broccoli into the baking dish. Pour heavy cream over broccoli then top with parmesan cheese, gruyere cheese, and mozzarella cheese.

4.Select Bake mode. Set time to 10 minutes and temperature 375 F then press START.

5.The air fryer display will prompt you to ADD FOOD once the temperature is reached then place the baking dish in the air fryer basket. Serve and enjoy

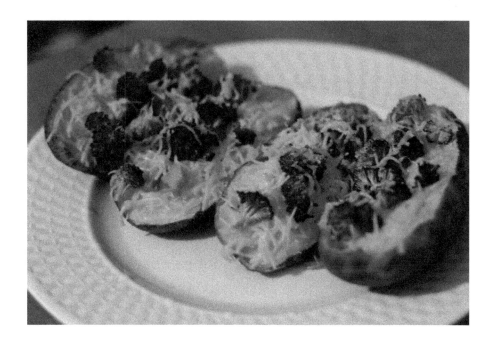

Stuffed Bell Peppers

Preparation Time:

10 minutes

Cooking Time:

45 minutes

Serve: 4

Ingredients:

4 eggs
2 medium bell peppers, sliced in half and remove seeds
1/2 cup parmesan cheese, grated
1/2 cup mozzarella cheese, shredded
1/2 cup ricotta cheese
1/4 cup baby spinach
1/4 tsp dried parsley
1 tsp garlic powder

Directions:

1.Add three cheeses, parsley, garlic powder, and eggs in food processor and process until combined.

2.Pour egg mixture into each pepper half and top with baby spinach.

3.Place stuffed peppers in a baking dish. Cover dish with foil. Select Bake mode. Set time to 45 minutes and temperature 375 F then press START.

4.The air fryer display will prompt you to ADD FOOD once the temperature is reached then place the baking dish in the air fryer basket. Serve and enjoy.

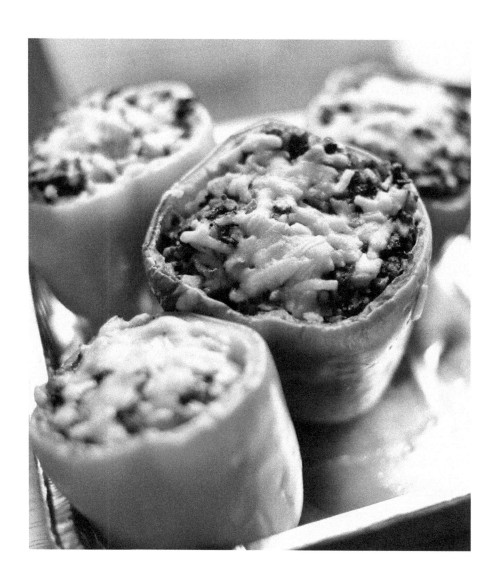

Delicious Zucchini Casserole

Preparation Time:

10 minutes

Cooking Time:

30 minutes

Serve: 6

Ingredients:

3medium zucchini, sliced into

1/4-inch thick slices

1 tbsp butter

2 tbsp unsweetened almond milk

1/3 cup heavy cream

3 oz brie cheese

1/2 tbsp Italian seasoning

1 cup Swiss gruyere cheese, shredded

2 garlic cloves, minced

Pepper Salt

Directions:

1.Toss zucchini slices with salt and place into a colander and set aside for 45 minutes.

2.Pat dry with a paper towel. In a baking dish, arrange zucchini slices and season with pepper and salt.

3.Combine brie, garlic, butter, almond milk, and cream

in a small saucepan and heat for few minutes or until cheese melts.

4.Pour cheese mixture over zucchini and sprinkle with shredded cheese. Top with Italian seasoning. Select Bake mode. Set time to 30 minutes and temperature 400 F then press START.

5.The air fryer display will prompt you to ADD FOOD once the temperature is reached then place the baking dish in the air fryer basket. Serve and enjoy.

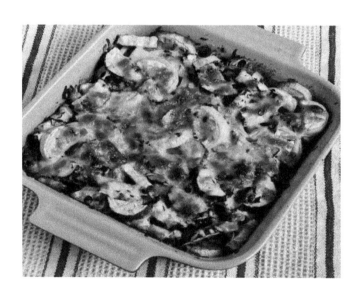

Parmesan Squash Casserole

Preparation Time:

10 minutes

Cooking Time:

45 minutes

Serve: 4

Ingredients:

3medium squash, cut into slices

1/4 cup parmesan cheese, shredded

3/4 stick butter, cut into cubes

1 medium onion, sliced

Pepper Salt

Directions:

1.Layer slices squash, onion, butter, pepper, and salt. Sprinkle with shredded parmesan cheese in a baking dish. Cover dish with foil.

2.Select Bake mode. Set time to 45 minutes and temperature 350 F then press START.

3.The air fryer display will prompt you to ADD FOOD once the temperature is reached then place the baking dish in the air fryer basket. Serve and enjoy.

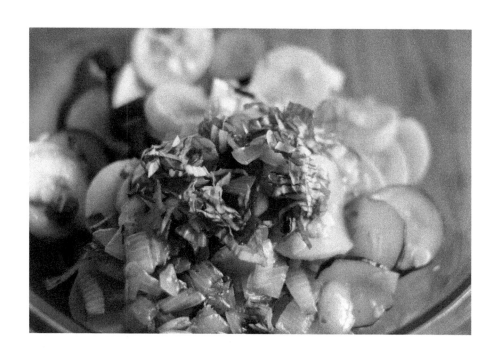

Pecan Green Bean Casserole

Preparation Time:

10 minutes

Cooking Time:

20 minutes

Serve: 4

Ingredients:

1 lb green beans, trimmed and cut into pieces
1/4 cup olive oil
2 oz pecans, crushed
1 small onion, chopped
2 tbsp lemon zest
1/4 cup parmesan cheese, shredded

Directions:

1.Add all ingredients into the mixing bowl and toss well. Spread green bean mixture into the baking dish.

Select Bake mode.

2.Set time to 20 minutes and temperature 400 F then press START. The air fryer display will prompt you to ADD FOOD once the temperature is reached then place the baking dish in the air fryer basket. Serve and enjoy

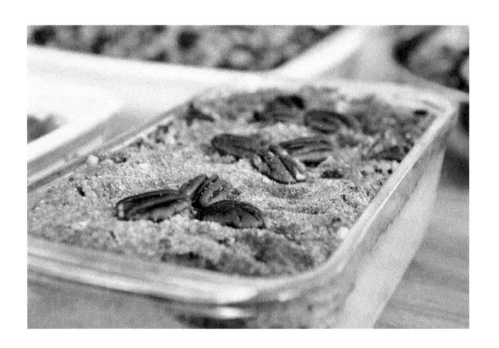

Brussels Sprouts and Broccoli

Preparation Time:

10 minutes

Cooking Time:

30 minutes

Serve: 6

Ingredients:

1 lb broccoli, cut into florets
1 lb Brussels sprouts, cut ends
1 tsp paprika
1/2 onion, chopped
1 tsp garlic powder
1/2 tsp pepper
3 tbsp olive oil
3/4 tsp salt

Directions:

1.Add all ingredients into the mixing bowl and toss well. The spread vegetable mixture in a baking dish. Select Bake mode.

2.Set time to 30 minutes and temperature 400 F then press START. The air fryer display will prompt you to ADD FOOD once the temperature is reached then place the baking dish in the air fryer basket. Serve and enjoy

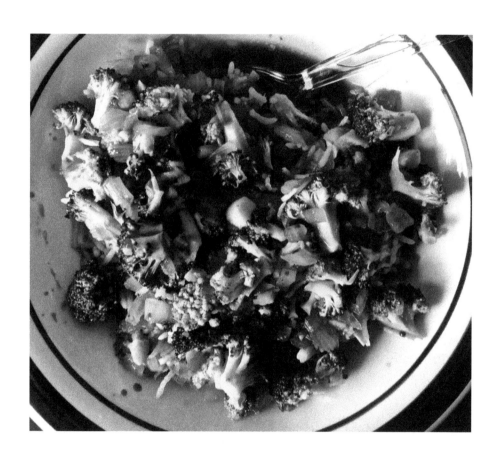

Basil Eggplant Casserole

Preparation Time:

10 minutes

Cooking Time:

35 minutes

Serve: 6

Ingredients:

1 eggplant, sliced
3 zucchini, sliced
4 tbsp basil, chopped
1 tbsp olive oil
3 garlic cloves, minced
3 oz mozzarella cheese, grated
1/4 cup parsley, chopped
1 cup grape tomatoes, halved
1/4 tsp pepper
1/4 tsp salt

Directions:

1.Add all ingredients into the large bowl and toss well to combine. Pour eggplant mixture into the greased baking dish.

2.Select Bake mode. Set time to 35 minutes and temperature 350 F then press START.

3.The air fryer display will prompt you to ADD FOOD once the temperature is reached then place the baking dish in the air fryer basket.

Serve and enjoy.

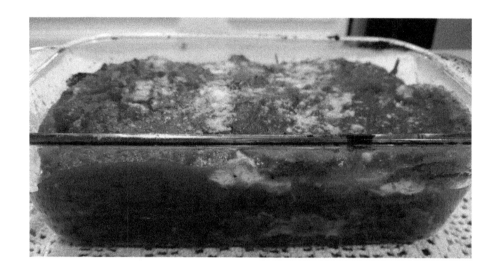

Spicy Okra

Preparation Time:

10 minutes

Cooking Time:

10 minutes

Serve: 2

Ingredients:

1/2 lb okra, trimmed and sliced
1 tsp olive oil
1/8 tsp pepper
1/2 tsp chili powder
1/2 tsp garlic powder
1/4 tsp salt

Directions:

1.Add all ingredients into the bowl and toss well. Select Bake mode.

2.Set time to 10 minutes and temperature 350 F then press START.

3.The air fryer display will prompt you to ADD FOOD once the temperature is reached then add okra in the air fryer basket. Stir halfway through. Serve and enjoy.

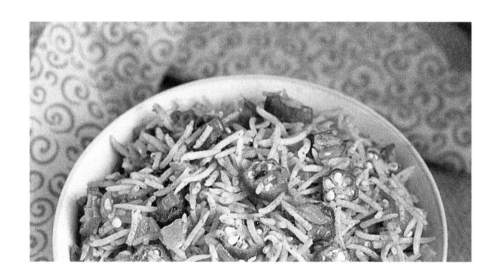

Air Fry Asparagus

Preparation Time:

10 minutes

Cooking Time:

10 minutes

Serve: 4

Ingredients:

1lb asparagus, ends trimmed and cut in half

1 1/2 tbsp coconut aminos

2 tbsp olive oil

1 tbsp vinegar

Pepper Salt

Directions:

1.Add asparagus in a large bowl with remaining ingredients and toss well.

2.Select Air Fry mode. Set time to 10 minutes and temperature 400 F then press START.

3.The air fryer display will prompt you to ADD FOOD once the temperature is reached then place asparagus in the air fryer basket. Stir halfway through. Serve and enjoy.

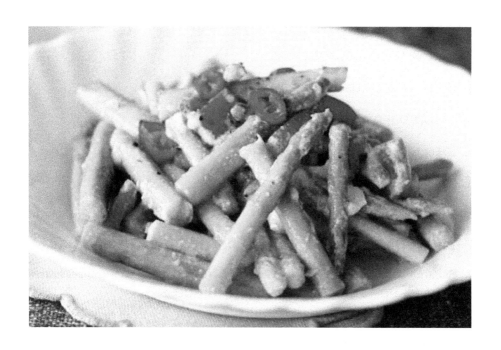

Crisp Brussels Sprouts

Preparation Time:

10 minutes

Cooking Time:

15 minutes

Serve: 4

Ingredients:

1cups Brussels sprouts

1/4 cup almonds, crushed

1/4 cup parmesan cheese, grated

2 tbsp olive oil

2 tbsp everything bagel seasoning

Salt

Directions:

1.Add Brussels sprouts into the saucepan with 2 cups of water. Cover and cook for 8-10 minutes.

2.Drain well and allow to cool completely. Sliced each Brussels sprouts in half.

3.Add Brussels sprouts and remaining ingredients into the mixing bowl and toss to coat. Select Air Fry mode. Set time to 15 minutes and temperature 375 F then press START.

4.The air fryer display will prompt you to ADD FOOD once the temperature is reached then add Brussels sprouts mixture in the air fryer basket. Serve and enjoy.

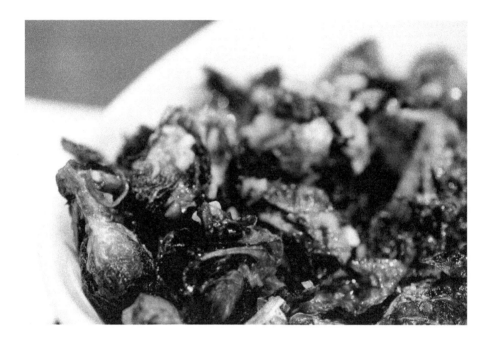

Tasty Cauliflower Rice

Preparation Time:

10 minutes

Cooking Time:

40 minutes

Serve: 8

Ingredients:

6 cups grated cauliflower
1/8 tsp red pepper flakes
2 tbsp fresh cilantro, chopped
10 oz can tomatoes with green chilis
1/2 tsp salt

Directions:

1.Add can tomatoes into the blender and blend well. Add grated cauliflower, cilantro, tomatoes, red pepper flakes, and salt into the prepared baking dish and stir until well combined.

2.Select Bake mode. Set time to 40 minutes and temperature 350 F then press START.

3.The air fryer display will prompt you to ADD FOOD once the temperature is reached then place the baking dish in the air fryer basket. Serve and enjoy.

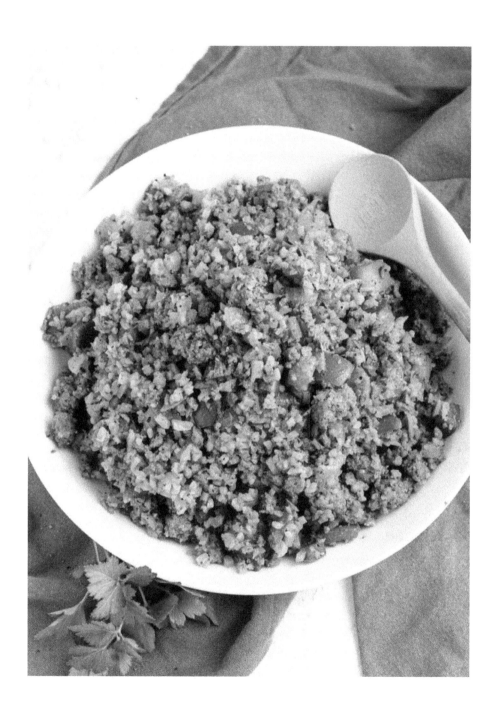

87

Spinach Squares

Preparation Time:

10 minutes

Cooking Time:

35 minutes

Serve: 9

Ingredients:

3 eggs
1/2 cup ricotta cheese
16 oz frozen spinach, cooked and drained
8 oz cheddar cheese, grated
1/2 tsp paprika
Pepper Salt

Directions:

1.Add eggs, paprika, ricotta cheese, pepper, and salt into the blender and blend until smooth. Stir in spinach and cheese.

2.Pour egg mixture into the greased baking dish. Select Bake mode.

3.Set time to 35 minutes and temperature 350 F then press START.

4.The air fryer display will prompt you to ADD FOOD once the temperature is reached then place the baking dish in the air fryer basket. Slice and serve.

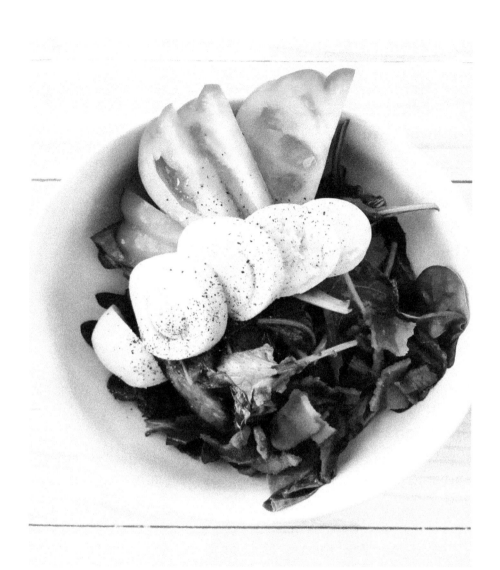

Vegetable Kebabs

Preparation Time:

10 minutes

Cooking Time:

10 minutes

Serve: 4

Ingredients:

2 bell peppers, cut into
1-inch pieces
1 eggplant, cut into
1-inch pieces
1/2 onion, cut into
1-inch pieces
1 zucchini, cut into
1-inch pieces
Pepper Salt

Directions:

1.Thread vegetables onto the soaked wooden skewers and spray them with cooking spray. Season with pepper and salt.

2.Select Air Fry mode. Set time to 10 minutes and temperature 390 F then press START.

3.The air fryer display will prompt you to ADD FOOD once the temperature is reached then place skewers in the air fryer basket. Turn halfway through. Serve and enjoy.

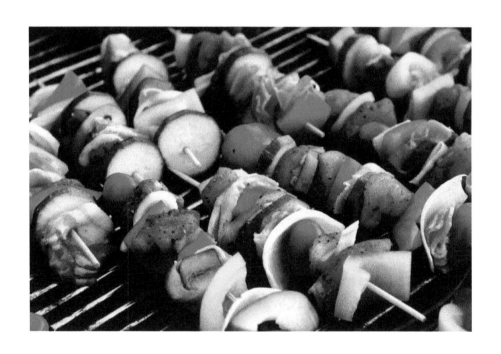

Old Bay Calamari

Cook Time:

20 minutes + Marinating Time

Servings:3

Ingredients:

1cup beer

1 pound squid, cleaned and cut into rings

1 cup all-purpose flour

2 eggs

1/2 cup cornstarch

Sea salt, to taste

1/2 teaspoon ground black pepper

1 tablespoon Old Bay seasoning

Directions:

1.Add the beer and squid in a glass bowl, cover and let it sit in your refrigerator for 1 hour. Preheat your Air Fryer to 390 degrees F.

2.Rinse the squid and pat it dry. Place the flour in a shallow bowl.

3.In another bowl, whisk the eggs. Add the cornstarch and seasonings to a third shallow bowl. Dredge the calamari in the flour.

4.Then, dip them into the egg mixture; finally, coat them with the cornstarch on all sided. Arrange them in the cooking basket.

5.Spritz with cooking oil and cook for 9 to 12 minutes, depending on the desired level of doneness. Work in batches. Serve warm with your favorite dipping sauce. Enjoy!

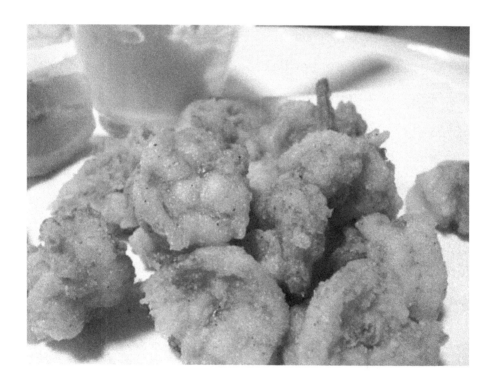

Grilled Tilapia with Portobello Mushrooms

Cooking Time:

20 minutes

Servings:4

Ingredients:

1tilapia fillets

1 tablespoon avocado oil

1/2 teaspoon red pepper flakes, crushed

1/2 teaspoon dried sage, crushed

1/4 teaspoon lemon pepper

1/2 teaspoon sea salt

1teaspoon dried parsley flakes

4medium-sized Portobello

1mushrooms
A few drizzles of liquid smoke

Directions:

1.Toss all ingredients in a mixing bowl; except for the mushrooms. Transfer the tilapia fillets to a lightly greased grill pan.

2.Preheat your Air Fryer to 400 degrees F and cook the tilapia fillets for 5 minutes. Now, turn the fillets over and add the Portobello mushrooms.

3.Continue to cook for 5 minutes longer or until mushrooms are tender and the fish is opaque. Serve immediately. Enjoy!

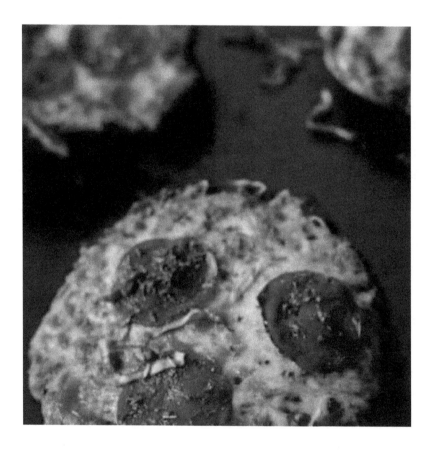

Crunchy Topped Fish Bake

Cook Time:

20 minutes

Servings: 3

Ingredients:

1 tablespoon butter, melted

1 medium-sized leek, thinly sliced

1 tablespoon chicken stock

1 tablespoon dry white wine

1 pound tuna

1/2 teaspoon red pepper flakes, crushed

Sea salt and ground black pepper, to taste

1/2 teaspoon dried rosemary

1/2 teaspoon dried basil

1/2 teaspoon dried thyme

2 ripe tomatoes, pureed

1/4 cup breadcrumbs

1/4 cup Parmesan cheese, grated

Directions:

1.Melt 1/2 tablespoon of butter in a sauté pan over medium-high heat. Now, cook the leek and garlic until tender and aromatic.

2.Add the stock and wine to deglaze the pan. Preheat your Air Fryer to 370 degrees F. Grease a casserole dish with the remaining 1/2 tablespoon of melted butter. Place the fish in the casserole dish.

96

3.Add the seasonings. Top with the sautéed leek mixture.

4.Add the tomato puree. Cook for 10 minutes in the preheated Air Fryer.

5.Top with the breadcrumbs and cheese; cook an additional 7 minutes until the crumbs are golden.Serve and enjoy!

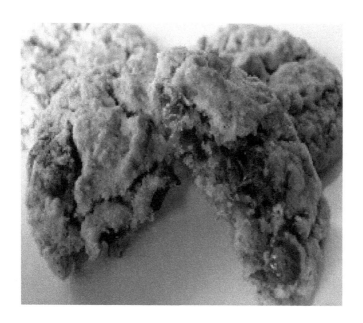

Beer Battered Fish with Honey Tartar Sauce

Cook Time:

20 minutes

Servings:2

Ingredient

1/2 pound hoki fillets

Sea salt and black pepper, to taste

1/2 cup flour

1 egg

1 teaspoon paprika

1 12-ounce bottle beer

1/4 cup mayonnaise

1/2 teaspoon honey

1 tablespoon fresh lemon juice

1 teaspoon Dijon mustard

1 teaspoon sweet pickle relish

Directions:

1.Rinse the hoki fillets and pat dry. Combine the flour, egg and paprika in a bowl.

2.Gradually pour in beer until a batter is formed. Dip the fish fillets into the batter; then, transfer to the lightly greased cooking basket.

3.Cook in the preheated Air Fryer at 380 degrees F for 12 minutes.

4.In the meantime, whisk the remaining ingredients to make the sauce. Place in the refrigerator until ready to serve. Enjoy!

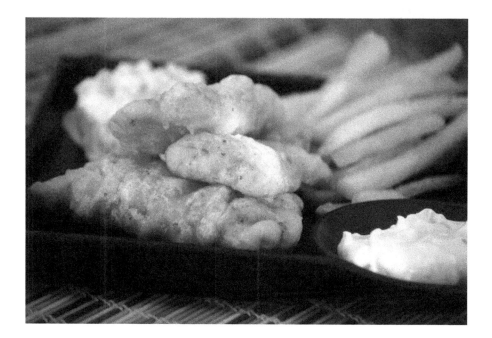

Snapper with Coconut Milk Sauce

Cook Time:

20minutes

Servings:2

Ingredients:

1/2 cup full-fat coconut milk

2 tablespoons lemon juice

1 teaspoon fresh ginger, grated

2 snapper fillets

1 tablespoon olive oil

1 tablespoon cornstarch

Salt and white pepper, to taste

Directions*:*

1.Place the milk, lemon juice, and ginger in a glass bowl; add fish and let it marinate for 1 hour.

2.Removed the fish from the milk mixture and place in the Air Fryer basket. Drizzle olive oil all over the fish fillets.

3.Cook in the preheated Air Fryer at 390 degrees F for 15 minutes.

4.Meanwhile, heat the milk mixture over medium-high heat; bring to a rapid boil, stirring continuously.

5.Reduce to simmer and add the cornstarch, salt, and pepper; continue to cook 12 minutes more. Spoon the sauce over the warm snapper fillets and serve immediately.

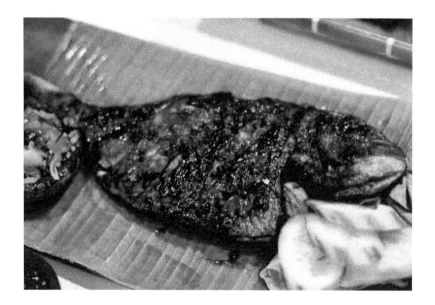

Moroccan Harissa Shrimp

Cook Time:

10 minutes

Servings:3

Ingredients:

1pound breaded shrimp, frozen

1 teaspoon extra-virgin olive oil

Sea salt and ground black pepper, to taste

1 teaspoon coriander seeds

1 teaspoon caraway seeds

1 teaspoon crushed red pepper

1 teaspoon fres garlic, minced

Directions:

1.Toss the breaded shrimp with olive oil and transfer to the Air Fryer cooking basket.

2.Cook in the preheated Air Fryer at 400 degrees F for 5 minutes; shake the basket and cook an additional 4 minutes.

3.Meanwhile, mix the remaining ingredients until well combined. Taste and adjust seasonings. Toss the warm shrimp with the harissa sauce and serve immediately. Enjoy!

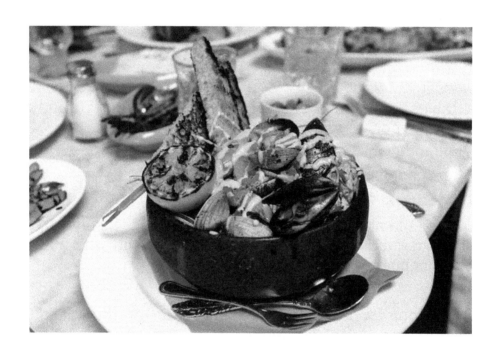

Anchovy and Cheese Wontons

Cook Time:

15 minutes

Servings:2

Ingredients:

½ pound anchovies

½ cup cheddar cheese, grated

1 cup fresh spinach

2 tablespoons scallions, minced

1 teaspoon garlic, minced

1 tablespoon Shoyu sauce Himalayan salt and ground black pepper, to taste

½ pound wonton wrappers

1 teaspoon sesame oil

Directions:

1.Mash the anchovies and mix with the cheese, spinach, scallions, garlic and Shoyu sauce; season with salt and black pepper and mix to combine well.

2.Fill your wontons with 1 tablespoon of the filling mixture and fold into triangle shape; brush the side with a bit of oil and water to seal the edges.

3.Cook in your Air Fryer at 390 degrees F for 10 minutes, flipping the wontons for even cooking. Enjoy!

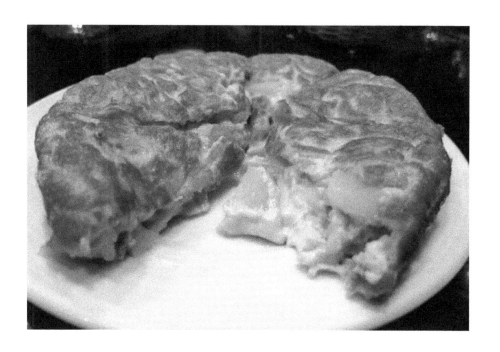

Seed-Crusted Codfish Fillets

Cook Time:

15 minutes

Servings:2

Ingredients:

1codfish fillets

1 teaspoon sesame oil

Sea salt and black pepper, to taste

1 teaspoon sesame seeds

1 tablespoon chia seeds

Directions:

1.Start by preheating your Air Fryer to 380 degrees F. Add the sesame oil, salt, black pepper, sesame seeds and chia seeds to a rimmed plate.

2.Coat the top of the codfish with the seed mixture, pressing it down to adhere.

3.Lower the codfish fillets, seed side down, into the cooking basket and cook for 6 minutes. Turn the fish fillets over and cook for a further 6 minutes. Serve warm and enjoy!

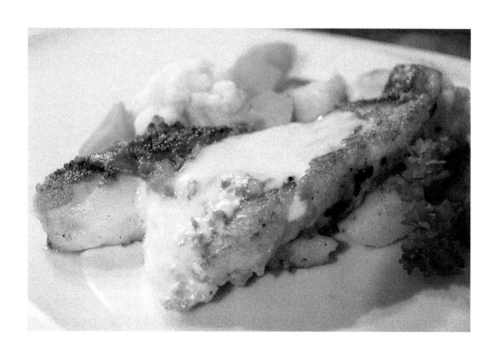

Tuna Steaks with Pearl Onions

Cook Time:

20 minutes

Servings:4

Ingredients:

4 tuna steaks

1 pound pearl onions

4 teaspoons olive oil

1 teaspoon dried rosemary

1 teaspoon dried marjoram

1 tablespoon cayenne pepper

1/2 teaspoon sea salt

1/2 teaspoon black pepper, preferably freshly cracked

1 lemon, sliced

Directions:

1.Place the tuna steaks in the lightly greased cooking basket.

2.Top with the pearl onions; add the olive oil, rosemary, marjoram, cayenne pepper, salt, and black pepper. Bake in the preheated Air Fryer at 400 degrees F for 9 to 10 minutes.

3.Work in two batches. Serve warm with lemon slices and enjoy!

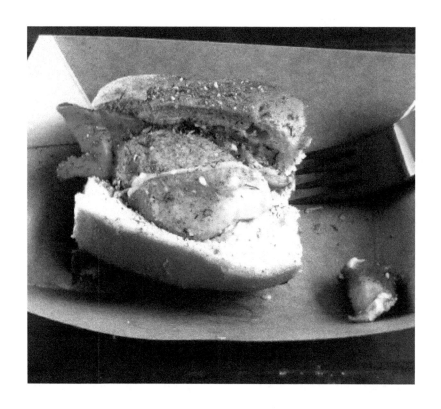

English-Style Flounder Fillets

Cook Time:

20 minutes

Servings:2

Ingredients:

2 flounder fillets

1/4 cup all-purpose flour

1 egg

1/2 teaspoon Worcestershire sauce

1/2 cup bread crumbs

1/2 teaspoon lemon pepper

1/2 teaspoon coarse sea salt 1/4 teaspoon chili powder

Directions:

1.Rinse and pat dry the flounder fillets. Place the flour in a large pan.

2.Whisk the egg and Worcestershire sauce in a shallow bowl.

3.In a separate bowl, mix the bread crumbs with the lemon pepper, salt, and chili powder. Dredge the fillets in the flour, shaking off the excess. Then, dip them into the egg mixture.

4.Lastly, coat the fish fillets with the breadcrumb mixture until they are coated on all sides. Spritz with cooking spray and transfer to the Air Fryer basket.

5.Cook at 390 degrees for 7 minutes. Turn them over, spritz with cooking spray on the other side, and cook another 5 minutes. Serve and enjoy!

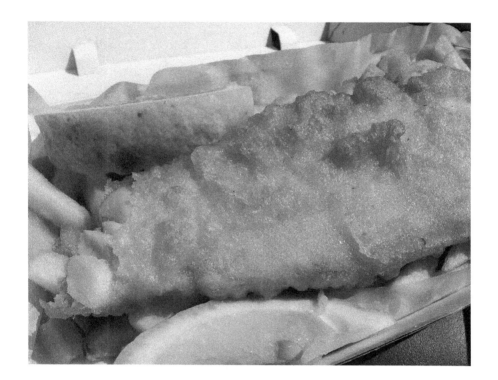

Lightning Source UK Ltd.
Milton Keynes UK
UKHW020713270521
384463UK00001B/75